CANNABIS
AND OTHER SUBSTANCE USE

An Information Guide for Adolescents

Anne Kwamie

Cannabis and Other Substance Use
Copyright © 2019 by Anne Kwamie

All rights reserved. No part of this
publication may be reproduced, distributed,
or transmitted in any form or by any means,
including photocopying, recording, or
other electronic or mechanical methods,
without the prior written permission of
the author, except in the case of brief
quotations embodied in critical reviews
and certain other non-commercial
uses permitted by copyright law.

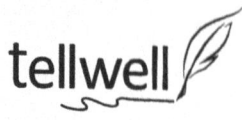

Tellwell Talent
www.tellwell.ca

ISBN
978-0-2288-1007-0 (Paperback)
978-0-2288-1009-4 (eBook)

Dedicated to the glory of God.
To Yosef, Aku and Nana Asante,
for your love and support

Table of Contents

Acknowledgements 1
Introduction 3

A. All About Cannabis 4
   Cannabinoids 5
   History of Cannabis Use in Canada 5
   Safety of Cannabis in Canada 6

B. Cannabis Use and the Law 7
   Legal Cannabis Use in Canada 7
      Recreational Cannabis and the Law 8
      Medicinal Cannabis and the Law 8
   The Cannabis Act and Adolescents 9

C. How Cannabis and Other Substances Are Used ... 11
   Cannabis Use 11
      Recreational Cannabis 11
      Medicinal Cannabis 12
   Other Substance Use 13

D. Cannabis and Your Health 15
   How does the Adolescent Brain Work? 15
   Effects of Cannabis and Other Substances
   on Adolescent Health 18

- Harmful Effects of Cannabis and Other Substances 19
- Tolerance and Dependency 24
  - Tolerance 24
  - Dependency and Addiction 25
- How to Tell if You Are Dependent on Substances 26
- Myths About Cannabis Use 27
- How to Tell if You Are at Risk for Substance Use 28

E. Resisting Substance Use 29
- Know Your True Self 29
  - The Power to Resist Substance Use: Testing Your Will 30
  - Staying in Control 33
  - Uplifting Activities 33
- Getting Help 37
  - Where to Go for Support 37
  - National 37
  - Alberta 38
  - British Columbia 38
  - Manitoba 39
  - New Brunswick 39
  - Newfoundland and Labrador 39
  - Northwest Territories 40
  - Nova Scotia 40

    Nunavut 41
    Ontario 41
    Prince Edward Island 42
    Quebec 42
    Saskatchewan 43
    Yukon 43
F. Did You Know…? 43
G. If You Are Using: Be Safe! 44

References 47
Glossary 53
About the Author 57

Acknowledgements

This health promotion booklet and the information within it would not have become a reality but for the kind assistance and review of these dedicated and supportive health care professionals, who I would like to thank:

Dr. L.D. Thomson, MD FCFP
Assistant Professor
Department of Paediatrics, Queen's University (Rtd)

Dr. Martin A. Katzman, BSc, MD, FRCPC
Clinic Director, START Clinic for
Mood and Anxiety Disorders
Research Director (Dean), Department of
Psychology, Adler Graduate Professional School
Northern Ontario School of Medicine

Introduction

As an adolescent, you may have been exposed to others who use cannabis, and you might have tried it yourself. In 2015, and again in 2017, a Health Canada survey from the Canadian Tobacco Alcohol and Drugs Survey (CTADS) estimated that 25% of young people in Canada used cannabis. This means that one in four Canadian youth used cannabis, second only to alcohol. Another study, by the World Health Organization in 2016, confirmed that cannabis use by Canadian youth was the second highest in the world, while a United Nations study in 2016 identified Iceland as the country with the highest use of cannabis by people aged 15 years and above.

Concerns about the high use of substances among youth are global. Recent reports from the U.S. Food and Drug Administration (FDA, 2018) express concerns about a significant increase in substance use with innovative vaping devices among high school students. Similarly, health care providers in Canada worry about adolescents' increased use of substances and their risk of accidental overdose.

According to Statistics Canada, the legalization of recreational cannabis in Canada is likely to lead adolescents to increase their use. There will also likely be a lot of discussion amongst adolescent peer groups on social media about the legalization and availability of cannabis, and adolescents are also expected to try new products or purchase cannabis from illicit sources.

The aim of this booklet is to give adolescents current information on cannabis and other substances. The booklet also seeks to help adolescents understand the laws around cannabis and how it is used. It then explains the harmful effects that regular use of cannabis and other substances can have on adolescents' health. Finally, this booklet invites you to consider the benefits of drug-free living by suggesting ways to resist substance use, including a list of resources across Canada where you can find support.

A. All About Cannabis

Cannabis is a complex plant that is also known by different street names, including *marijuana*, *pot*, *weed*, *hash*, *honey oil*, *phoenix tears*, and *shatter*. It grows mainly in tropical countries and in structured, warm environments. The cannabis plant contains over 100 different complex chemicals, some of which are not well understood. The complex chemicals are found in the flowering tops and leaves of the cannabis plant. These complex chemicals are called *cannabinoids*.

Cannabinoids

The main cannabinoid in cannabis is known as THC (-delta 9 tetrahydrocannabinol). The next most plentiful cannabinoid is cannabidiol, or CBD, which is non-stimulating, so it is preferred for medicinal purposes.

THC produces the "high" sensation and intoxication of cannabis, along with other effects. CBD's effects are opposite to those of THC. It produces a calm, muted effect and decreases THC's intoxicating or high effect. The potency of cannabis depends on the ratio of THC to CBD. Research studies into using CBD to treat diseases are ongoing. THC has been studied extensively and has been found to have the highest concentration in the dried, matured flowering tops of the cannabis plant.

History of Cannabis Use in Canada

Historically, Canadians have used cannabis for leisure and relaxation since the early 1900s. It is believed to have been introduced to North America from India. Initially, cannabis was used for treating various illnesses and was widely available over the counter in local pharmacies.

Medicinal cannabis use decreased as more effective, scientific-based medicines became available, but recreational use continued. Throughout the mid-1900s, medical scientists determined that using cannabis for relaxation was harmful because it affected people the same way that narcotics such as opium did (Houlihan, 2016). They petitioned to have cannabis listed as a controlled drug. As a result, a law was passed in Canada in 1923, making cannabis use illegal — one of many countries in the world to do so (UNODC, 2016).

In spite of the introduction of this law, people continued to use cannabis illegally, for leisure and relaxation. During the 1960s, recreational cannabis use became more popular, and Canadians, including young people, have continued to possess and use cannabis to this day, even though it had been illegal to do so until recently.

Safety of Cannabis in Canada

Health Canada is leading the way to safeguard the quality of cannabis and its legalization in Canada. Authorized producers, distributors, and growers of cannabis are supervised and expected to meet strict standards. These standards ensure that the cannabis produced in Canada is of high quality; safe; and free of insecticides, bacteria, and fungus. As a result of these strict standards, Canadians can be confident that the cannabis they purchase and use from authorized vendors is safe.

In spite of Health Canada's strict rules and regulations that make it safer to use, there are still risks when using low quality and dangerous forms of cannabis. For example, synthetic marijuana, known as a type of "designer drug," has been available on the Canadian black market since 2000 and is increasingly available to Canadians. These designer drugs are prepared to have similar chemical qualities and effects as the THC found in the natural cannabis plant. Synthetic cannabinoid brands on the market may be known by other names, such as "K2" or "Spice." "Spice" is an herb that has been spiked or sprayed with synthetic cannabinoids to produce a similar high, along with other mood-altering effects of cannabis. Synthetic marijuana is sometimes labelled as "herbal incense" or "herbal smoking blends." These brands may be deadly and are illegal worldwide.

B. Cannabis Use and the Law

Legal Cannabis Use in Canada

Currently, there are two ways that cannabis is used legally in Canada — recreationally and medicinally — and the laws are different for each category.

Recreational Cannabis and the Law

Recreational cannabis refers to the use of cannabis for leisure or relaxation. Recreational cannabis use was legalized in Canada in October 2018, making it lawful and available to Canadians over the age of 18, who are now free to grow, possess, and buy cannabis for their personal use from licensed retailers or facilities.

Medicinal Cannabis and the Law

Medicinal cannabis, also referred to as "cannabis for medical purposes," has been legal in Canada since 2001. Some people with chronic illnesses use cannabis to relieve symptoms that are not helped by regular treatments or prescription medications. Some people with illnesses or conditions such as multiple sclerosis, epilepsy, sleep disorders, cancer, and chronic pain have said they experienced improvement and relief from their symptoms with cannabis use. Medicinal cannabis makes it possible for Canadians to improve their medical conditions and have a better quality of life.

Initially, people who were authorized to use cannabis medicinally could use it only in its dried form. However, in 2015, a Supreme Court ruling allowed licensed producers to expand their product lines to include cannabis oil, fresh cannabis buds, and leaves. Edibles such as brownies, candy, and cookies made from these products are also now available for medical purposes.

People using medicinal cannabis need a prescription from their doctor or nurse practitioner. This health care practitioner first does a thorough assessment of the patient's medical condition before authorizing medicinal cannabis use. Then, the patient is able to get quality-controlled cannabis by registering with licensed producers and Health Canada. Regulations allow people to grow their own cannabis or appoint someone else to grow it for them. These people are limited to a 30-day supply of cannabis at a time.

The Cannabis Act and Adolescents

Canadians, including adolescents, have commonly used cannabis or marijuana for leisure over the years. However, it has been unlawful to do so until recently. On October 17, 2018, the Government of Canada passed the *Cannabis Act*, which makes recreational use of high-quality cannabis legal for Canadians in all provinces and territories. The *Cannabis Act* is federal legislation that protects the health and safety of Canadians by ensuring that harmful cannabis is not available for use. There are rules that control the way cannabis is produced, distributed, sold, and possessed in Canada. This act relates only to recreational cannabis use.

The *Cannabis Act* clearly states that recreational cannabis use in Canada is legal only for adults — adolescents are not allowed to have or use cannabis. **It is unlawful and a crime for youth under 18 years of age to have or use cannabis for recreation.** This means that Canadian youth should not purchase, use, or have cannabis on their person. It is also a crime for an adolescent to have a grow-op or to give another person permission to have, grow, import, or export cannabis on their behalf.

The *Cannabis Act* was passed, after a debate, to protect the health and safety of Canadians by legalizing recreational cannabis use. Illegal sales of harmful and poor-quality cannabis for recreational use had become very lucrative in Canada, and this new law ensures the quality of cannabis sold. This law also protects adolescents, by preventing them from getting cannabis and by making it illegal for advertisers to package and label cannabis products that are appealing to youth.

Only authorized or licensed producers and retailers are allowed to produce, distribute, and sell cannabis to Canadians. Adult users are allowed to grow up to four plants for their own personal use. Cannabis in food and beverages is allowed for medicinal use but not for recreational use, at this time. Cannabis sales are currently available online and will be available through authorized storefronts and other retail facilities in 2019, in all provinces and territories except Nunavut.

ALERT: The new Canadian law legalizes the recreational use of cannabis for adults only. IT REMAINS A CRIME FOR ADOLESCENTS TO HAVE, USE, OR SELL CANNABIS! (Minimum age for recreational use of cannabis is 18 or 19 years, depending on the province or territory).

C. How Cannabis and Other Substances Are Used

Cannabis Use

Recreational Cannabis

People use recreational cannabis in a variety of forms to achieve the desired effects or high. These are some of the forms in which it can be used:

- ROLLED CIGARETTES: Cannabis may be smoked in the form of a rolled cigarette known as a *joint*. The average joint contains approximately 0.5 to 1.0 gram of dried cannabis.
- PIPE OR BONG: It can also be smoked in a pipe or filtration device known as a *bong*. Pipes are used to smoke dried cannabis, which is either

tightly packed solid or in a sticky paste called *resin* (also known as *hash*). Smoked cannabis works rapidly to provide a high within minutes. Cannabis smoke contains many of the chemicals found in tobacco smoke, but cannabis smoke is harsher on the lungs. The THC content in hash can be potent — hash resin can contain up to 65% THC, while the content in hash oil is between 30 and 90%.
- VAPING: Cannabis can be inhaled with a vaporizer or an e-cigarette device. This process is known as *vaping*. Public health institutions are concerned about the increase in the number of adolescents who are vaping.
- EDIBLES: The sale of cannabis in the form of foods and beverages is not currently allowed for recreational use.

Medicinal Cannabis

For medicinal purposes, cannabis can be used in all the forms above as well as these forms:

- EDIBLES: Cannabis can be made into "edibles'" or food, like cookies, candy, or brownies, and beverages like teas.
- CANNABIS OIL: Cannabis oil can be used in skin creams, butters, oils, and ointments, as

well as compresses. THC is absorbed easily through the skin into the bloodstream to provide the desired effect.
- CAPSULES AND TABLETS: Cannabis is also available in capsule and tablet forms.

People taking these forms of cannabis for medicinal purposes experience the additional effects of cannabis differently, depending on their medical condition and the nature and form of cannabis they are taking.

Other Substance Use

Cannabis is identified as a substance. *Substances* are chemicals that can cause harm to the brain and change how the brain works. **When you use cannabis, you are using a substance.**

In addition to cannabis, you may come across other substances that are readily available on the street. These street drugs can cause harm to your brain when used together with cannabis. All substances, including cannabis, can be abused or cause intoxication. These are some of the other substances adolescents might come across:

- HALLUCINOGENIC DRUGS: Hallucinogenic drugs cause excitement and hallucinations.

PCP (phencyclidine or "angel dust") and LSD ("acid") are examples of hallucinogens.
- INHALANTS: Inhalants are substances that are inhaled or sniffed through the nose or mouth. Paint thinners, glue, and aerosol spray are examples of inhalants.
- SEDATIVES AND TRANQUILIZERS: Sedatives and tranquilizers are substances that calm people down when they are anxious or agitated. Valium, Nembutal, Rohypnol ("roofies"), and Xanax are examples of sedatives and tranquilizers.
- STIMULANTS: Stimulants make the user more active, or "hyper." Cocaine, amphetamines, "uppers," "meth," and MDMA ("ecstasy" or "molly") are examples of stimulants. MDMA ("meth" or "ecstasy") has a higher risk of abuse.
- OPIOIDS: Opioids are narcotic painkillers. Increasing use of opioids is responsible for the current crisis of overdose deaths in Canada and other parts of the world. Opioids include heroin, fentanyl, codeine, Percocet, Percodan, and oxymorphone (Opana). Fentanyl is the most common street drug responsible for most overdose deaths in Canada.
- TOBACCO, ALCOHOL, AND OVER-THE COUNTER MEDICATIONS: Tobacco, alcohol,

and some over-the-counter medications like cold medicines are also considered substances. Using these substances can cause harmful effects on adolescent brain function.

Mixing substances like cannabis or opioids with alcohol can be deadly. This combination has been found to be responsible for suicides and accidental overdose deaths.

In 2017, the Canadian Centre on Substance Use and Addiction reported that more Canadians were using illegally obtained opioids than ever before. It was estimated that 4000 Canadians died from opioid overdose that same year. Overdose deaths from illegally obtained painkillers have become a public health crisis in Canada (Fischer, Pang, & Tyndall, 2018).

D. Cannabis and Your Health

How does the Adolescent Brain Work?

Your brain is the control centre of your performance and behaviour. It is responsible for your ability to think, remember, reason, feel, move, hear, see, taste, smell, and talk. A normal, highly functioning brain determines your character, emotions, intellect, and ability to understand and speak a language.

Adolescents who regularly use cannabis and other substances harm their physical and mental health. Studies show that substance use is harmful to the adolescent brain. The term *substance use* refers to regular consumption of substances such as alcohol, cannabis, tobacco, opioids, sedatives, stimulants, and over-the-counter medication. Scientific evidence also suggests a relationship between cannabis use in adolescents and the development of mental disorders such as psychosis. **Adolescents who avoid using substances reduce the risks to their health. They are also able to function at their overall best.**

Like the brains of adults, adolescents' brains are made up of complex networks of billions of nerve cells and fibres. These nerve cells and fibres receive and send signals between the brain and the body. This network enables your brain to exchange messages that allow it to organize body movements, stability, and other functions. The brain continues to grow and develop throughout the adolescent period and does not fully mature until the mid-30s.

During puberty, there is an imbalance in the body's systems due to the new release of hormones. Adolescents' behaviours and emotions are influenced by these hormones in the body. During this period of development, adolescents crave pleasure and engage in behaviours that produce excitement and relaxation to satisfy their pleasure-seeking ways.

The brain's reward centre is very active during this time, and adolescents seek to reward themselves with activities, situations, and objects that produce pleasure. They take pleasure in making new friends and establishing meaningful relationships with others. Some adolescents become defiant or engage in risky sports activities, like extreme or adventure sports. Adolescence is also a time when you develop the ability to make decisions, perform well at school, and learn to control your impulses. During healthy adolescence, behaviour and personality are a part of normal growth and development.

During this period when the brain reorganizes and matures, adolescents are at particular risk of being influenced by their surroundings. The maturing brain is easily affected and harmed by substances during this time, and using those substances can lead to mental problems, right away or later on in adulthood. Several studies, including one by Jacobus and Tapert (2014), show that **cannabis use by adolescents can cause permanent harm to the structure of the brain and the young person's ability to think, learn, understand, reason, and remember things.** Adults are better able than adolescents to withstand the harsh effects of cannabis because of the maturity of the adult brain.

Effects of Cannabis and Other Substances on Adolescent Health

Each adolescent experiences the effects of substance use differently because each person is different. There are several factors that change the way each person is affected by cannabis and other substances:

- AGE: Taking cannabis together with other substances affects adolescents and adults differently, and the effects are more intense for adolescents.
- PRE-EXISTING CONDITIONS: Pre-existing medical and psychological conditions can also influence the effects of cannabis.
- ENVIRONMENT: The environment in which cannabis is used can intensify its effects.
- AMOUNT, FREQUENCY, AND FORM: The amount of the substance used, how often it is used, and the type and strength of the substance all influence its effects.

Recreational cannabis affects users in a variety of ways. It can bring on feelings of joy, ecstasy, euphoria, relaxation, excitement, and being in "seventh heaven."

Here are some details about the timing of the effects of cannabis:

- Effects are felt within fifteen minutes of smoking or inhaling and are known as the marijuana "high."
- The effects can be short-lived or last for several hours.
- Smoking or vaping cannabis has immediate effects, while eating cannabis products results in a slower high but a more long-lasting effect.
- THC stays in fat cells of the body for anywhere from days to weeks before the body gets rid of it, and it is therefore easy to detect on drug tests.

Harmful Effects of Cannabis and Other Substances

If you currently use cannabis and other substances, or have been using them for a while, you should know how these substances can negatively affect and harm you. Research studies on adolescents show increasing evidence of a connection between the use of cannabis and other substances and the development of mental disorders. This includes suicidal thoughts, suicide attempts, and following through with suicide.

The harmful effects of substance use interfere with normal adolescent development, including physical, psychological, and social changes.

- COMBINATION EFFECT: **Combining cannabis with other substances can cause harm and accidental death.**

  - If cannabis is taken regularly together with alcohol, illegal drugs, prescription drugs, over-the-counter cold medications, or herbal products, users experience dangerous and more powerful effects.
  - Cocaine and cannabis taken together can cause chest pain or a heart attack within one hour of use.
  - Opioids or tranquilizers taken together with alcohol can result in death by overdose.

- SYNTHETIC CANNABINOIDS: **Using synthetic cannabinoids or using cannabis together with other substances are both extremely unsafe and hazardous to an adolescent's health and well-being.**

- Synthetic cannabinoids, known as "Spice" or "K2," can cause seizures, palpitations, psychosis, schizophrenia, and death.
- Inhalants like paint thinners and glue can cause cancer, memory loss, psychosis, and death.
- Using PCP can result in seizures, low blood sugar, and coma.
- Heavy ecstasy users can experience high blood pressure, stroke, muscle pain, bowel infection, movement impairment, and dental decay known as "meth mouth."

- CHANGES IN BEHAVIOUR: Using cannabis can lead to changes in behaviour, including the following:

  - Shamelessness, bold attitudes, increased hunger, excessive social media activities, and excessive time spent watching videos or gaming
  - Relaxation, loud talking or giggling/laughter
  - Tension, anxiety, aggravation, fear, confusion

- Decreased energy, decreased ambition, poor judgement, risky sexual behaviour, or trouble with the law

- CHANGES IN BRAIN DEVELOPMENT: Using cannabis can lead to changes in brain development, including the following:

  - Inability to think straight, inability to remember or reason, and poor performance at school
  - Short attention span, impaired ability to drive or operate machinery, drowsiness, and mental clouding
  - With heavy use, difficulty concentrating and retaining information
  - A warped sense of time and a sense of being "stuck"

- CHANGES IN BRAIN FUNCTION: Changes in brain function can include depression, psychosis, and a variety of mental disorders. Researchers note that when adolescents regularly use cannabis and other substances, this can lead to mental disorders such as first episode schizophrenia and other psychoses. Schizophrenia is the most common form of psychosis that can affect vulnerable adolescents who use cannabis. It can occur suddenly or slowly, in the late teens or early twenties. People with schizophrenia may lose touch with reality and be unable to communicate or relate to others. Other symptoms of psychosis are hallucinations, delusions, and disorganized thoughts and speech. Timely treatment after the first episode can have positive results, improve symptoms, and allow the person to live independently. Symptoms may remain for life, but some adolescents recover completely with early treatment.

- CHANGES IN PHYSICAL WELL-BEING: Using cannabis can lead to changes in physical well-being, including the following:

  - Red eyes, feeling sick, vomiting, dry mouth and throat, dizziness, inability to speak clearly, weakness, palpitations, dullness, sluggishness, and clumsiness.
  - With prolonged use, abdominal pain, menstrual cycle changes, and suppression of ovulation in women; low libido, and problems with sperm health in men.

- Decline in physical activity and possible reduction in immune system function.

- CHANGES IN SOCIAL WELL-BEING: Using cannabis can lead to changes in social well-being, including the following:

  - Loneliness, an inability to make friends, poor relationships with others, and dissatisfaction with self.
  - Dropping out of school, low self-esteem, poor communication and social skills, unemployment, criminal behaviour, difficulties with work or school, and managing daily affairs.

Tolerance and Dependency

Tolerance

Over time, regular users of a substance develop tolerance to that substance. Someone experiencing *tolerance* to a substance needs to use more of it to achieve the same desired effect. Tolerance can be reversed, and the need for more of the substance can wear off quickly after the person stops using the substance. **Adolescents who regularly use cannabis**

and other substances risk developing tolerance to those substances.

Dependency and Addiction

Adolescents are using recreational cannabis and other substances in increasing numbers. Several studies show that adolescents who use cannabis regularly risk becoming dependent on it or addicted to it. The terms *dependency* and *addiction* are used interchangeably to describe a more serious problem than tolerance. A person is described as dependent on or addicted to a substance when the cravings are out of control and the person continues to use the substance despite being aware of the harmful effects. People who use substances heavily over a long period of time can become addicted to or dependent on those substances. They need to continuously use the substance, and the need is urgent to prevent withdrawal symptoms.

When the substance a person is dependent on is not available, is stopped abruptly, or is reduced in dose, the person may experience withdrawal symptoms. These symptoms show up in physical or psychological ways and can occur within one or two days of the person being without that substance.

Someone experiencing withdrawal symptoms may experience the following:

- Emotional changes such as anger, anxiety, restlessness, irritability, or depression
- Disturbed sleep, nightmares, or strange dreams
- Decreased appetite, weight loss, or cravings
- Headaches, red eyes, high blood pressure, or chest pain

It is extremely important to seek immediate medical attention during the withdrawal period for managing this dangerous health situation. Most symptoms will settle down within one to two weeks of treatment. **Research studies have shown that when adolescents use substances — including cannabis — at an early age, they are highly likely to become addicted to those substances (CCSA, 2017).**

How to Tell if You Are Dependent on Substances

You are considered dependent on or addicted to cannabis or other substances when you experience at least two of the following signs within one year:

- You are unable to perform regular tasks, like going to school or work.

- You continue to use substances in risky situations, like interacting with drug dealers.
- You are unable to cut down on substance use no matter how hard you try.
- You continue to crave and use a particular substance even though you know it has a negative impact on your existing medical condition.
- You have reached tolerance level to the substance — you need to use more to get the same effect.
- You are experiencing some withdrawal symptoms.
- You spend a lot of time looking for, using, and recovering from using a substance.
- You have abandoned activities you previously loved doing and spend more time using substances.
- You continue to use substances despite the negative effects this has on your relationships.

Myths About Cannabis Use

Myths about cannabis use are widespread. Many adolescents have beliefs about cannabis that are untrue. The following statements are examples of myths about cannabis:

- Cannabis use does not harm you.
- You cannot get addicted to cannabis.
- Cannabis is not as popular as other drugs.
- There are no long-term consequences to cannabis use.
- You cannot overdose on cannabis.

How to Tell if You Are at Risk for Substance Use

Not all adolescents use or want to start using substances, but some are more likely to start than others. Adolescents at higher risk for substance use are those who:

- Are vulnerable to peer pressure
- Seek to reward themselves with pleasurable activities
- Feel disrespected by or disappointment from their parents (most adolescents wish to be respected and trusted by their parents)
- Come from homes with little or no supervision
- Live in deprived communities or environments that make life unpleasant, lonely, boring, or dull
- Come from families that are poorly educated and have low-income

- Are depressed, socially and geographically isolated, and unemployed
- Associate with people who are delinquent, use substances, and have behavioral problems
- Have low self-esteem
- Are bullied at school, face racism, or are snubbed by peers
- Are from a dysfunctional home environment, where parents or other adults use substances
- Are stressed by unrealistic expectations placed on them
- Live with existing physical or mental health conditions

E. Resisting Substance Use

Know Your True Self

The World Health Organization describes adolescence as a period of life between the ages of 10 and 19 (WHO, 2018). During this period of development, young people try to steer their way into adulthood as their bodies go through physical, intellectual, personality, social, and psychological changes. Adolescence is that time of life when young people gain qualities and abilities that allow them to enjoy their youth and assume adult roles later on. Adolescents become vibrant, cheerful, enthusiastic, optimistic, affectionate, confident, outgoing, curious, joyful, and full of life and energy. They also become self-centred and attention-seeking, as they seek to establish their identity and independence. **Well-adjusted adolescents are happy people.**

During this period of development, adolescents establish meaningful relationships, make new friends easily, and are excited about dating. They are hungry to find new interests and possibilities in life. They love to explore what the world has to offer in amusement or inspiration and gain new knowledge and skills. They learn to make decisions and control their impulses. As adolescents achieve normal biological growth and development, they become aware of their true selves. **The adolescent years are exciting — a time when adolescents enjoy their lives and look forward to successful education and career opportunities in the future.**

The Power to Resist Substance Use: Testing Your Will

Healthy adolescents have principles and qualities that make them self-confident, sociable, and able to solve problems. They can own these qualities to help fight back and overcome the temptation that can drive them toward substance use. Adolescents need encouragement to boost emotions that promote happiness. Happy people are successful in terms of social and work relationships, friendships, finances, independence, life satisfaction, and well-being. Confident adolescents are aware of their true self qualities. They are satisfied with themselves and are familiar with the health risks of substance use. As a result, substance use becomes an unattractive non-starter. Adolescents who are aware of their true selves have the power and self-control to turn down offers to try cannabis and other substances.

As an adolescent, you have qualities that can help you resist substance use, and you can test your will to resist substances by focusing on the following:

- You are able to resist peer pressure and resist acting in ways to please others.
- You have ethical personal standards that you act and live by.
- You are able to find and take advantage of opportunities in the environment you live in.
- You control and manage everyday affairs and situations effectively.
- You are aware that you are continuing to improve as you grow and develop as a person.
- You are open to new experiences that interest you and are not bored with life.

- You recognize that you are able to contribute positively to society.
- You have a sense of self-control and can say "no thanks" when offered substances.
- You know yourself and the world around you.
- You feel you are always growing and developing new attitudes and behaviours.
- You enjoy warm, open, satisfying relationships with others.
- You show concern for the welfare of others.
- You understand the give and take of human relationships and make compromises to maintain ties to others.
- Your goals in life have a sense of direction.
- You understand that life has meaning, so you have aims and objectives for living.
- You have a positive view of yourself and your past experiences.
- You accept personal qualities, good and bad.
- You are happy with who you are.

If you are not using cannabis or other substances, don't start. If you are thinking about trying cannabis and other substances, make sure you first get the information you need about substance use and the health risks involved. Better still, abstain! Don't start! If you are curious and want to try using cannabis, do your best to delay doing so until later in life.

Staying in Control

Adolescents can live happy, successful, meaningful lives by rejecting cannabis and other substance use when they try these things:

- Overcome personal problems and difficulties
- Be highly productive in your community
- Overcome difficulties like unemployment, loneliness, social isolation, low self-esteem, a dysfunctional home environment, and dissatisfaction with life.
- Seek counselling and participate in uplifting activities.

Uplifting Activities

Uplifters are activities that can do the following:

- Boost adolescents' emotional, financial, and social well-being.
- Give a natural buzz that helps adolescents feel upbeat, optimistic, stress-free, resilient, and competent.
- Boost adolescents' energy and self-esteem.

- Stimulate stronger relationships with others, and help adolescents to be more engaged in their communities.
- Promote better adjustment at school.

Uplifting activities involve a higher participation in hobbies, team sports, new experiences, creative pursuits, and leisure activities. They help adolescents realize their inner strength and ability to live a meaningful and purposeful life.

Here are some ideas for uplifting activities:

- Reduce screen time — spend less time on social media, texting, gaming, watching TV, and Internet surfing.
- Spend more time in person-to-person interaction.
- Make friends with people who look different from you.
- Spend more time with friends.
- Participate in school sports and physical fitness.
- Participate in spiritual activities.
- Watch the sunrise and sunset, every now and then.
- Volunteer at a community centre, school, hospital, or farm.

- Carry out a random act of kindness.
- Complete a 1,000-piece puzzle.
- Make a scrapbook with memories of your school year.
- Start a savings account.
- Get skills training and employment through community youth programs.
- Learn to cook.
- Plan to study in a different country.
- Visit a museum.
- Learn about other cultures.
- Explore and learn about Indigenous people of Canada.
- Participate in a powwow, at least once.
- Learn a new language.
- Express your thoughts and feelings through paint on canvas.
- Appreciate natural beauty and quiet spaces.
- Surround your personal space with memorable items, plants, and wood-crafted items.
- Create a visual image of your dreams and life goals — DAYDREAM.
- Experience life without TV, Internet, phone, or radio for 24 hours.
- Be a tourist in your own town or city.
- Love life. Be thankful.

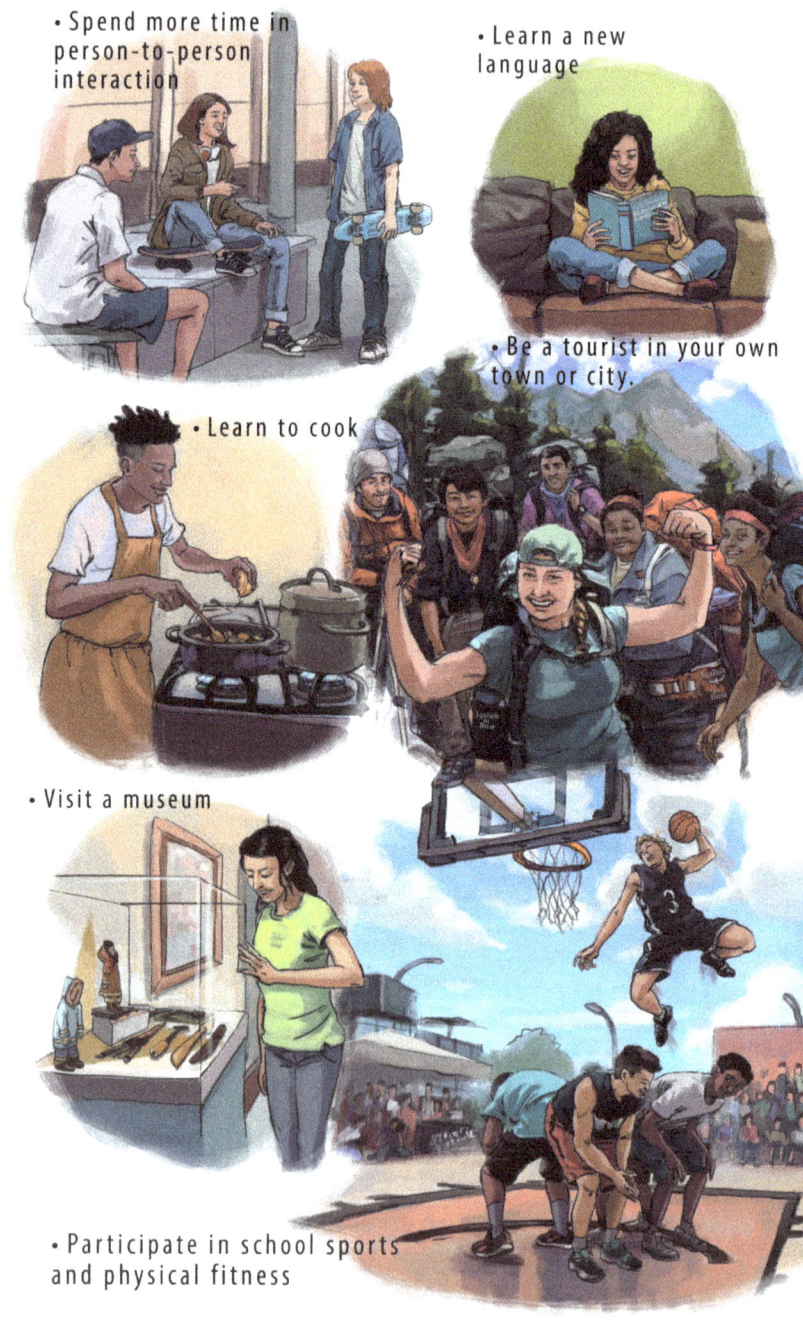

Getting Help

Where to Go for Support

If you need to discuss and reduce the negative consequences of substance use, seek professional help. Help is readily available in all Canadian provinces and territories.

Talk to your parents, a community elder, or trusted adult if you are exposed to, overwhelmed by, or pressured to use substances. Often, parents are more understanding than adolescents might think they are.

Visit your health care provider for professional help. Health care providers are available in community health centres, family health teams, nurse practitioner–led clinics, nursing stations, health posts, and Aboriginal health access centres. Physicians and nurse practitioners in these facilities can provide health care services and connect you to appropriate professional services in the community for counselling.

National

- Kids Help Phone: 1-800-668-6868 (open 24 hours), www.kidshelpphone.ca

- Canadian Centre on Substance Use and Addiction (CCSA): www.ccdus.ca
- Drug Free Kids Canada: https://www.drugfreekidscanada.org
- Canadian Association of Mental Health (CAMH): https://www.camh.ca/
- Youth Canada: https://www.canada.ca/en/services/youth.html
- Health Care Services for First Nations and Inuit: https://www.canada.ca/en/indigenous-services-canada/services/health-care-services-first-nations-and-inuit.html

Alberta

- Health Link: 811 or 1-866-408-5465 (open 24 hours), www.healthlink@albertahealthservices.ca
- Mental health helpline: 1-877-303-2642 (open 24 hours)
- ConnecTeen: 1-403-264-TEEN(8336), https://calgaryconnecteen.com, ConnecTeen@distresscentre.com

British Columbia

- Health Link: 811 (open 24 hours)
- HealthLink BC: https://www.healthlinkbc.ca/

- Kelty Mental Health Resource Centre: https://www.keltymentalhealth.ca
- Foundry: https://www.foundrybc.ca

Manitoba

- Health Links/Info Santé: 211 or 1-204-788-8200, https://misericordia.mb.ca/health-links-info-sante-phcc/
- First Nations and Inuit Hope for Wellness Help Line: 1-855-242-3310
- Manitoba Addictions Helpline (Youth): 1-877-710-3999, http://mbaddictionhelp.ca/services/addiction-services-for-youth/

New Brunswick

- Tele-Care: Patient Connect NB: 811, https://www2.gnb.ca/content/gnb/en/departments/health/Tele-Care.html
- Partners for Youth: 1-506-462-0323, http://www.partnersforyouth.ca/en/

Newfoundland and Labrador

- Health Links: 811 (open 24 hours), https://www.yourhealthline.ca/links

- Youth Mental Health Counsellor: 1-709-777-2200
- Canadian Mental Health Association Newfoundland and Labrador: https://cmhanl.ca

Northwest Territories

- NWT Help Line: 1-800-661-0844 (open 24 hours)
- Mental Health and Addictions: https://www.hss.gov.nt.ca/en/services/mental-health, mha@gov.nt.ca
- Health and Social Services Community Counselling: https://www.hss.gov.nt.ca/en/contact/community-counsellor

Nova Scotia

- Help Line: 811 Peace of mind (open 24 hours)
- Nova Scotia Health Authority (health care providers): www.nshealth.ca

Nunavut

- Kamatsiaqtut Help Line: 1-867-979-3333, http://www.nunavuthelpline.ca/
- Department of Health (information): 1-867-975-5700

Ontario

- Youth Employment Services (YES): https://www.yes.on.ca
- First Nations and Inuit Hope for Wellness Help Line: 1-855-242-3310 (open 24 hours/7 days a week)
- Aboriginal Health Access Centres: https://www.aohc.org/aboriginal-health-access-centres
- Community Health Centres: https://www.aohc.org/community-health-centres
- Nurse Practitioner-Led Clinics: https://www.aohc.org/nurse-practitioner-led-clinics/
- Family Health Teams: http://www.health.gov.on.ca/en/pro/programs/fht/
- Health Care connect: 1-800-445-1822 (open 24 hours), http://www.health.gov.on.ca/en/ms/healthcareconnect/pro/
- Connex Ontario: Addiction, Mental Health, and Problem Gambling Treatment

Services: 1-866-531-2600 (open 24/7), www.connexontario.ca

Prince Edward Island

- Telehealth 811: 811 (open 24 hours), https://healthpei.ca/811
- The Island Helpline for Mental Health Services: 1-800-218-2885, https://www.princeedwardisland.ca/en/information/health-pei/call-island-helpline
- Patient Registry Program: 1-855-563-2101 (toll-free), https://www.princeedwardisland.ca/en/information/health-pei/patient-registry-program

Quebec

- Info-Sante 811: 811 (open 24 hours), https://www.quebec.ca/en/health/finding-a-resource/consult-a-professional/info-sante-811/
- Action on Mental Illness (Agir contre la maladie mentale) (AMI-Québec): 514-486-1448,
- https://amiquebec.org
- Local Community Service Centre (CLSC): www.sante.gouv.qc.ca/repertoire-ressources/clsc/

Saskatchewan

- HealthLine: 811 (open 24 hours), https://www.saskatchewan.ca/residents/health/accessing-health-care-services/healthline
- Child and Youth Community Mental Health Services Community Care Branch: 1-306-787-7239, https://www.saskatoonhealthregion.ca/locations services/Services/mhas

Yukon

- Yukon HealthLine 811: 811 (open 24 hours), http://www.hss.gov.yk.ca/811.php
- Health Centres: www.hss.gov.yk.ca/healthcentres.php
- Mental Wellness and Substance Use Services: www.hss.gov.yk.ca/mwsu.php

F. Did You Know…?

- Opioids and over-the-counter cough and cold medicines are the most commonly abused substances after marijuana and alcohol.
- Alcohol use is harmful to your health.
- Alcohol consumption kills more than three million people, mostly men, each year,

according to the World Health Organization (WHO, 2018).
- Worldwide, people 15 years of age and over drink an average of 6.2 litres of alcohol every year (WHO, 2018).
- Adolescents who abuse prescription drugs are often given these drugs by friends or family members.
- Regular use of substances can lead to failure in school or at work.
- Tobacco (cigarettes) is a substance, and its use is responsible for the death of half of its users (WHO, 2018).
- Engaging in healthy leisure activities can help develop self-worth, self-control, and social connectedness.
- Half of adolescents' waking life is available for leisure.
- Problematic use of social media has the potential to be addictive.
- Problematic use of Facebook can lead to anxiety and depression (Marino, Gini, Vieno, & Spada, 2018).

G. If You Are Using: Be Safe!

You can reduce the most harmful effects of cannabis by following these rules:

- Don't use synthetic cannabinoids like "Spice" or "K2" — they can be deadly.
- Choose safer methods of cannabis use.
- If you smoke, avoid harmful smoking practices like smoking in enclosed spaces or passing off second-hand smoke to others.
- Limit how much cannabis you use and how often you use it.
- If you use cannabis, don't drive or operate any machinery.
- If you are at risk for a mental health disorder or are pregnant, avoid cannabis use altogether.

References

Bradley, G.L., & Inglis, B.C. (2012). Adolescent leisure dimensions, psychosocial adjustment, and gender effects. *Journal of Adolescence, 35*, 1167–1176.

Canadian Centre on Substance Abuse (CCSA). (2017). *Canadian youth perceptions on cannabis.* Retrieved from http://www.ccsa.ca/Resource%20Library/CCSA-Canadian-Youth-Perceptions-on-Cannabis-Report-2017-en.pdf.

Canadian Centre on Substance Use and Addiction. (2017). *Canadian drug summary: Prescription opioids.* Retrieved from http://www.ccsa.ca/Resource%20Library/CCSA-Canadian-Drug-Summary-Prescription-Opioids-2017-en.pdf.

Canadian Tobacco Alcohol and Drugs (CTADS). (2015). *2015 Summary.* Retrieved from https://www.canada.ca/en/health-canada/services/canadian-tobacco-alcohol-drugs-survey/2015-summary.html.

Cundiff, J.M, Kamarck, T.W., & Manuck, S.B. (2016). Daily interpersonal experience partially explains the association between social rank and physical health. *Annals of Behavioural Medicine, 50*, 854–861.

Fischer, B., Pang, M., & Tyndall, M. (2018). The Opioid death crisis in Canada: Crucial lessons for public health (Comment). *The Lancet*. Retrieved from https://doi.org/10.1016/S2468-2667(18)30232-9.

Government of Canada. (2018). *Cannabis in Canada.* Retrieved from www.Canada.ca/Cannabis.

Government of Canada. (2018). *National report: Apparent opioid-related deaths in Canada.* Retrieved from https://www.canada.ca/en/public-health/services/publications/healthy-living/national-report-apparent-opioid-related-deaths-released-march-2018.html.

Government of Canada. (2018). The *Cannabis Act.* Retrieved from https://laws-lois.justice.gc.ca/eng/acts/C-24.5/.

Government of Canada. (2016). *Update on the Supreme Court of Canada Decision in R. V. Smith- Canada.* Retrieved from https://www.

canada.ca/.../update-supreme-court-canada-decision-smith-health-canada.

Houlihan, B. (2016). Sir. William Brooke O'Shaughnessy — Medical cannabis pioneer. *Medium.* Retrieved from https://medium.com>sir-william-brooke.

Jacobus, J., & Tapert, S.F. (2014). Effects of cannabis on the adolescent brain. *Curr Pharm Des.* 20(13), 2186–2193.

Lubans, D.R., Smith, J.J., Morgan, P.J., Beauchamp, M.R., Miller, A., Lonsdale, C., ... Dally, K. (2016). Mediators of psychological well-being in adolescent boys. *Journal of Adolescent Health, 58,* 230–236.

Marino, C., Gini, G., Vieno, A., & Spada, M.M. (2018). The associations between problematic Facebook use, psychological distress and well-being among adolescents and young adults: A systematic review and meta-analysis. *Journal of Affective Disorders, 226,* 274–281. doi:10.1016/j.jad.2017.10.007.

Rana, S., & Nandinee, D. (2016). Profile of adolescents' positive emotions: An indicator of their psychological well-being. *Psychological Studies, 61*(1), 32–39.

Statistics Canada. (2018). *National cannabis survey, Second quarter 2018.* Retrieved from https://www150.statcan.gc.ca/n1/daily-quotidien/180809/dq180809a-eng.htm.

United Nations Office on Drugs and Crime (UNODC). (2016).*World drug report 2016*. Retrieved from https://www.unodc.org/wdr2016/.

U.S. Food and Drug Administration. (2018). *FDA launches new campaign: "The real cost"; Youth E-cigarette prevention campaign.* Retrieved from https://www.fda.gov/TobaccoProducts/PublicHealthEducation/PublicEducationCampaigns/TheRealCostCampaign/ucm620783.htm.

World Health Organization (WHO). (2018). *Adolescent health.* Retrieved from www.who.int/topics/adolescent_health/en/.

Zeidner, M., & Olnick-Shemesh, D. (2010). Emotional intelligence and subjective well-being revisited. *Personality and Individual Differences, 48,* 431–435.

> "...THE DAYS OF OUR YOUTH ARE
> THE DAYS OF OUR GLORY"
> —Lord Byron

Be Awesome. Live well.

Glossary

Addiction: A condition in which a person loses control and repeats behaviours and activities in spite of their negative effects.

Adolescents: People between the ages of 10 and 19, according to the World Health Organization.

Cannabinoids: Complex chemicals found in the flowers and leaves of the cannabis plant. THC and CBD are cannabinoids.

Cannabidiol (CBD): A chemical in cannabis that counterbalances the effects of THC.

Cannabis: A complex plant containing hundreds of chemicals that act on the brain to change the way one feels. Commonly known as *marijuana*.

Delusion: A false belief about oneself and the world.

Depression: A mental health condition with symptoms of sadness, discouragement, and despair that lasts continuously for at least two weeks.

Hallucinations: An experience in which a person smells, feels, sees, tastes, or hears things that are not there.

Inhalants: Substances that produce vapours and a "high" when inhaled.

MDMA: 3,4-Methylenedioxymethamphetamine. Also known as "ecstasy" or "molly."

Mental health: Psychological and emotional well-being that allows a person to problem-solve, work, love, and relate well to others.

Psychosis: A condition that alters normal thinking, speaking, and behaviour.

Schizophrenia: A mental disorder that alters normal thinking, speaking, and behaviour.

Substance abuse: Substance use at least three to four times per week.

THC (delta-9-tetrahydrocannabinol): The most plentiful chemical in the cannabis plant and which is responsible for the "high" effect of cannabis.

Tolerance: The need to continuously increase the amount of a substance used in order to achieve the desired "high" or intoxication.

Withdrawal: Severe symptoms that occur when a substance is cut off or the dose is reduced.

Youth: People between the ages of 15 and 34, according to Statistics Canada.

About the Author

Anne Kwamie is a nurse practitioner consultant in Ontario, Canada. She has worked as a community-based nurse practitioner, where she provided clinical services to individuals of all ages within the community.

She has also worked extensively with at-risk youth in the community, reinforcing youth health through clinical care, education, empowerment, and integration of health services.

She currently owns Sima Health Consultancy, where she offers services in primary health care consultancy, health care professional training, education, and community health promotion.

www.ingramcontent.com/pod-product-compliance
Ingram Content Group UK Ltd.
Pitfield, Milton Keynes, MK11 3LW, UK
UKHW020246240426
12048UKWH00027B/1633